RUN
FASTER
RACE
BETTER

BY COACH STEPHANIE ATWOOD

The **Big Book** of Track

and Speed Workouts for

- Runners

- Triathletes

- Team Sports and

- All Athletes Who Want to Be

FAST!

Revised, Revamped,

and

Ready to Rock and Roll!

This book combines the two Kindle Books *Run Faster Race Better and Run Faster Race Even Better* into **One BIG BOOK** of Track and Speed Workouts

For 5K

10K

Half Marathon

Full Marathon

Triathlons

Team Sports

Written and Compiled by

Coach Stephanie Atwood M.A.

coachstephanie@gowowteam.com

Best Selling Author

Nationally Certified Coach

Award Winning Runner

US Track and Field

Road Runners Club of America

ISBN-13: 978-0615824970 (At Last The Best)
ISBN-10:0615824978

http://**www.GoWOWTeam.com**
http://**www.facebook.com/GoWOWTeam**
https://www.facebook.com/pages/RunFasterRaceBetter/

Dedication

This book is dedicated to my parents. They always believed in me and allowed me to keep trying, even when they had questions about my sanity.

I want to thank my Mom for her special "can do" attitude for everything she approached. I learned from her.

I want to thank my Dad for his encouragement of whatever I was involved in. He let me be me!

What more could any child ask for than parents who said to go ahead. They always put their full love behind me - every crazy time! - Stephanie Atwood

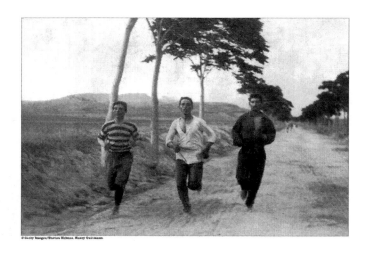

From the 1896 Olympic Marathon in Greece

Table of Contents

Foreword

As the adage goes, if you don't train fast then you can't race fast. OK - so I love to train fast, but then again, I know that it pays off with faster times and that feeling that I want. I know when I had a great workout. But sometimes it takes the help of the award winning, experienced, and trusted Stephanie Atwood to share just how to do that.

Speed training is a blend of science and art mainly because it is dependent on knowing your own tolerance - just how much and just how hard you can run in order to experience that wonderful magic of adaptation. Your muscles can and will adapt and contact faster, with more power.

So, the first point that you need to read about is that if you want to get faster, you have to include some (and hopefully just the right amount of) speed work to stimulate the adaptation process.

But there's more to it than just training fast. There's the next layer to successfully racing better. You need to know your pace and work out in a target area. Coach Stephanie, in her latest book on running, shares just how to know your pace, and shows you how to train yourself for that the target speed area that is optimum for you and your performance.

Training might seem as simple as lacing up the running flats and taking off fast and hard a couple of times a week , but if you do that , you are wasting valuable time, risking potential injury, and adding to the pile of junk miles. The solution? Variety.

This is the final key piece that Coach Stephanie will share with you in this great book - Run Faster, Race Better. I know after 40 years of racing, training, and prescribing running workouts, that a variety of workouts is key. By varying your daily workouts, you keep your mind and your body totally engaged and invigorated.

Varying workouts leaves no room for "same old, same old" complacency that keeps us from getting the results we seek. More of the same thing just leads to a type of training - monotony training - rather than variable training.

Make each of your run workouts more valuable than the one before. To accomplish this, do more than read Stephanie's new title - do everything she says and then watch the results. You will be able to do your best and after all, isn't that what you really want to accomplish?

Sally Edwards, MA, MBA
Founder and Developer of Heart Zones Training
Co-Author, *Be a Better Runner*
www.heartzones.com and www.zoningfitness.com

Introduction

When I first started running, we never ran on the track and speed work, as a term for long distance runners, may not have existed. That was a long time ago.

After I placed as the third woman in my first marathon, and knowing that I loved to compete, I decided to try my luck at track. I joined the community college team and started running laps. I was a miler and two miler before tracks went metric.

One of my main memories of that experience was how boring our workouts were. I ran 80 second laps, rested, then ran another 80 second lap, etc. all while the coach spent almost all of her time with the sprinters. I didn't know any better and loved to run. So, as a novice track competitor I did what I was directed to do.

Now many years later, as an experienced coach, I understand that my college coach had limited information (and maybe limited interests as well?) on how to help a distance runner improve with speed workouts.

Since endurance starts somewhere in the 800 – 1500m distance and just keeps going up to ultra-marathons, there are a many of us who can benefit from these workouts that focus on the aerobic energy system. Aerobic means we're using oxygen as the main compliment in our energy production.

I know speed workouts can help all runners improve. Speed work can help walkers too. I also know that the workouts themselves can vary and even be fun (in a painful kind of way). I developed three categories of workouts that can be used according to experience or periodization:

- **Least Hard**
- **Moderately Hard**
- **Hardest**

People with limited experience need to approach track with a conservative mind-set, and will want to start with the Least Hard workouts and move up from there. These workouts also fit in well for experienced runners who are in a maintenance period in their training or just need a "veg out" time on the track.

The Moderately Hard workouts can be used by anyone who has a good base. The minimum for a good base is 6 months of experience, exercising 3 times a week, running (or walking) a pace of 15 minutes or faster.

Clearly the runner who runs 5 minute miles is going to be doing the workout much differently than the walker who walks a mile in 15 minutes. Since the workouts are based on lap pace, both folks could be doing the same workout but their lap pace would be dramatically different. Interestingly however, the intensity for each person could be very similar. Intensity is measured by heart rate.

The Hardest category of workouts assumes that you have the base, endurance, and strength to complete an intense workout that generally lasts about 60 minutes total. This type of workout will build you up by breaking you down. You will be taxed to the max, given a rest, and then taxed again. This type of workout, for best effect, will require some rest time afterward for muscle recovery and improvement.

If you are doing hard, sustained workouts on the track, it is prudent (even if you are young) to give yourself time for your muscles to recover. It is in the recovery that we get stronger. My advice here is to do a hard workout followed by a day of cross training or all-out rest. Use different muscle sets on your cross training day or, if you are just too tired, don't do anything!

I have seen amazing improvement in people who do track workouts on a regular basis. The caveat is that it is easy to get injured if you overdo it. Listen to your body. Many forms of pain are not bearable and will only get worse if you ignore them.

Here are some terms to be aware of:
- Plantar fasciitis
- IT Band inflammation
- Stress fractures
- Knee pain
- Pulled psoas
- Tendonitis
- Sciatic Nerve

You may want to look these up if you already feel certain tweaks and twinges when you run.

Enjoy these workouts. I know, from working with my own clients and teams and from using them myself that they work for many different levels of ability and ages. Because there are so many, you could, if you choose, do a different one every week for the next year and then some.

Have fun, try hard, and tell me what you think by posting your questions on my Facebook page at www.facebook.com/gowowteam

Go for it!
Coach Stephanie

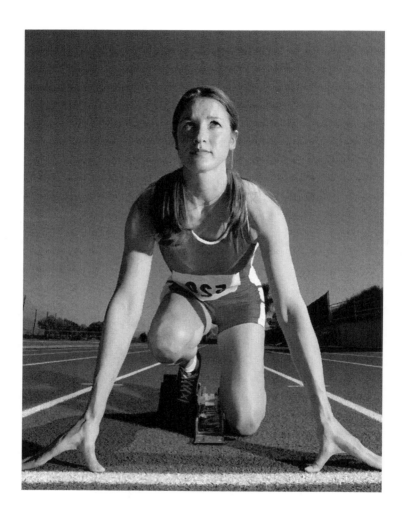

Perspective

In my first book on track workouts, I introduced the reader to the details of the track and touched on my experience with running over the past 30+ years. In those thirty years a lot of things have changed, and many for the good. Some of course have gone the other direction.

We have become a nation of runners. We exercise, we buy things, and we want the latest and best gadgets. And the market responds with more and more choices and better but often quite expensive equipment, programs, and tests to feed the beast.

Running used to be a sport where people trained and often raced in baggy shorts, cotton socks, Keds type clunker shoes, and clumsy, basic, cotton sweatshirts and warm-up pants. The fancy dressers wore polyester sweat suits. I had one for actual track meets. The track suit came after about 5 years of road running when I competed with a local college track team.

When I first started running, I was about 20 pounds heavier than I am now and determined that running after work, in the dark, would be a way to use up calories. I didn't tell anyone what I was doing and I sure didn't want them to see me out pounding the pavement. All my training was done at night. I started with one time around the block...Eventually I got up to enough times around one block that I expanded my boundaries.

Training for a marathon? Why not! I was young and had hiked 26 miles so let's give it a go!

I ran my first marathon in frumpy running shorts, cotton socks, Keds basketball type shoes, and a cotton t-shirt. Novice that I was, it shocked the heck out of me when I placed third woman! That was more than 30 years ago. I distinctly remember not being able to walk down stairs for several days following my victory and I don't remember my time. My last marathon gave me almost no muscle pain afterward at all and my time was good enough to qualify for the Boston Marathon with 27 minutes to spare. But, I digress...

Women didn't even have long distance running shoes formed for their feet at the time. I was lucky that my feet were wide, and once I learned that Keds were not the best shoe for marathons, I moved into men's shoes. There were a few brands and a few styles. They weren't then what they are now though. The prices, by 70's standards, were high and choice was low.

Training runs were all LSD (long, slow, distance) and none of us knew much about speed, nutrition, hydration, or any of it. Runner's World Magazine just started up around that time and we got race information from local running publications and word of mouth.

It was a different time. The field of runners was much smaller and, truthfully, more adjusted to the sport. They had to be a bit rough and determined because we didn't have the support that we have today. We just RAN! Literally, we ran every day (or almost). We ran far, if we could, for novices. I was putting in between 55 - 60 miles a week and doing almost nothing else to train. I loved it and it was what we thought was best for improving our running.

I think I was lucky to realize that, at 25, and not having graduated from college, I was eligible to run with the local college track team. I was just curious enough that I ended up at the track several times a week doing laps with the team. Today they would call this speed work. I just thought of it as fast running for short distances. It was hard but it made me a better road runner. Who would have guessed? Not I.

I got to be pretty good (for an older college student) at the 880 and mile distances. Tracks had not converted to metrics at that time. I learned a lot about competition, strategy, and absolute speed. I never was a sprinter, but I could hold my own in the mile and 2 mile races. It made me a better road runner and taught me about things like lactate threshold and "pushing through," though the science either wasn't there yet or my coaches weren't privy to that kind of information.

I also felt that the longer distances, for track, were pretty much looked down upon by the sprinters. I think it's still true today, to a great extent. Training for distance events, even 800's and up, takes time and a lot of running. Track training and speed workouts are not very social so the type of person who does the longer distance track races has to be able to handle the tedium and lack of social interaction, while being just as athletic and determined as the "fast twitch" sprinters who rarely run more than a 400 EVER!

Fast forward to 2013, I'm still doing laps at the track. I can see the difference that speed workouts make in my long distance running. Now I'm talking about 5K races and beyond. When you apply yourself at the track, you will get faster. I have documented this many times in my own training and with the runners I coach.

It is difficult to do track workouts. They are meant to be hard! The only time they should feel good is when they are over! But if you persist, YOU WILL GET FASTER! I highly recommend doing track workouts with a group or at least one other buddy. Misery seems to love company and there is something about working really hard that is better when it is shared.

One final word of advice before turning you loose to do the workouts. Speed work is the first thing that causes injury. Pushing yourself too hard without establishing a good base will set you up for injury. Approach the track gradually and not more than once a week. Maybe even once every two weeks in the beginning, as you build your overall running technique and strength.

If you start feeling pain that is more than just a short term sore muscle, pull back a bit. Those pulled muscles, inflamed joints, irritated tendons, and sensitive nerves are giving you a message that you're not quite ready for this new level of intensity. Be patient. Give your body time to adapt. Try again. Speed work is wonderful when you are ready for it.

The workouts I've written address different levels of ability, periods of training, and different states of health (injured and not). I have used them. My students and club members have used them. I believe in speed work when the time is right.

Have fun. Apply yourself. Go for it! - Coach Stephanie

Why Track?

I'm going to use this term lightly, because it also applies if you need to run somewhere besides on a track. Track, in a very general way of thinking, means fast to most runners. This is the way I use the term for this book. Track and speed are often times are synonymous in my definition.

What This Book Is

This book is a series of speed workouts that are often done on a track. The benefit of a track for speed type workouts is the ease of running a precise distance and allowing your mind and body to be fully committed to the workout. Tracks offer freedom from traffic, cracks in the pavement, dogs (for the most part) and other distractions to a great extent. They can give you the opportunity to focus specifically on the task at hand; and that task is usually speed.

You generally want to work at your calculated speed of 90% or above, depending on the purpose of the workout. I will discuss purpose and pace further on.

What This Book Is Not

This book is not for sprinters or runners who want to excel at a track competition. It does not focus on sprinters, and the anaerobic zone where they are often practicing. It does not focus on racing distances between 100m and 1500m or track competitions in general. If you run 5000m or 10000m on a track you can benefit from these workouts.

Yes, you can benefit from some of these workouts as soon as you get into aerobic type workouts; the main focus and purpose, however is to help endurance athletes who work out for durations farther than 1500 meters, longer than 10 seconds and all the way up to 50K's, maybe even a bit longer.

In addition to most endurance type running races, (2 mile, 5K, and up) this book would also apply to many field and team events where the meets could last for an hour or more where short bursts of speed may be essential to the competition and endurance for 30 minutes or longer may also be essential (soccer, rugby, lacrosse, baseball, crew, etc.).

The workouts are generally designed to take about 60 minutes to complete. Of course this depends on your running pace, and the number of sets. Feel free to adjust things to fit your own needs.

It is the intensity of the track workouts that offers such benefits. That same intensity (measured usually in speed) is what gets people injured. So, listen to your body and give yourself time to build up and solidify that base. Track workouts are meant to always be HARD.

When you apply yourself to that concept you will reap the benefits too. **You WILL improve!**

First Things First

Equipment

If you are prepared to work hard at the track, there is certain equipment that can really help you. If you don't have it, you are less able to control the workout. As Sally Edwards said in her book *Be A Better Runner*, there is a lot of technology and new science *"that can help people tap into the joy of running. And now, they finally want it"*.

Recommended Equipment

- Heart Rate Monitor
- Interval timer (Gymboss)
- Light weight (almost barefoot type) shoes
- Digital watch with easy readout
- Water bottle
- Healthy snack that steers clear of refined products and offers a pre and post workout ratio of 3:1 carbohydrate to protein (suggested possibilities - Larabar Uberbars, coconut water and nuts, or chocolate milk)

Track Etiquette

When you work out on the track there is definitely a protocol. Most of it is just plain common sense.

Inside lane = Lane #1. This is the fast lane. We all know this. However, there are two reasons to run in this lane and I want folks to understand both the etiquette and the common sense involved.

Etiquette says that the fastest runners get to train in this lane by virtue of their speed. What many novice runners don't realize initially is that the inside lane also offers the fastest circuit around the track.

It is a significant distance farther around the outside lane than running around the inside lane.

If you are serious about improving, and are pushing yourself to your personal limit during the workout, you also belong in this inside lane as long as there is no one faster barreling down on you. If that person is coming up on you please have the courtesy to move to your right.

Do this with enough time and after checking over your shoulder so that you don't have a whole pack of runners behind you. When and if that happens on the track, plan ahead, move out of their way, far to the right. Sometimes, however, you might just step to your left, off the track for a few seconds and this is best for the entire situation. Use your head and be aware.

I-pods or Music on the Track

I have seen too many inconsiderate people running or even walking on the inside lane with music playing so loudly that they are totally oblivious to what is happening around them. They definitely did not get the message.

Some people who are average sort of athletes, want to push themselves on the track and try to improve their speed. Please don't be one of those inconsiderate, unaware bodies on the track, hogging the inside lane. If you want to veg out, take the far right lane (Lane 8 usually) and do your thing.

This is a pet peeve of mine because I know how hard some folks want to push themselves. A thoughtless form, taking up space in lane one, adds an additional challenge that doesn't need to be there.

On the other hand, running around someone is not the end of the world. I try to keep it from making me lose my focus. So, in that way it can be used as a mental learning tool. I might be tempted to yell but don't want to use the energy. So be it...

Track workouts will cause you to SWEAT and raise your heart rate! If you have any reason why this is not wise, please make a good choice. We assume you have spoken with your doctor about exercising hard. Thank you!

Bring layers of clothing and water. There is usually no reason not to workout except for extreme weather. Be prepared. If the weather is cold or wet, have a change of clothes in your car or near-by. After the workout is when you get cold.

If the weather is really hot, bring water, a decent cap, sun screen and, if possible workout in the early morning, in shade, or later, when it cools down.

Guide to Terminology

Dynamic Stretches - There are different terms used in running and there are definitely different theories. What are dynamic stretches? These are active movements that you take before the main workout that complement the muscles that are used during the intense part of your exercise.

With running workouts, we want to warm up the legs, the arms, the shoulders, the hips, and the butt (the large muscle groups).   The reason? So that they are able to respond quickly to the forces put on them with the needed flexibility and power when we up the intensity.

Some suggested stretches include jumping jacks, hip rotations, skaters or cross overs, stationery bicycles (knees to alternate elbows), fast steps in place, striders. There are many. The purpose of 5 – 10 minutes of warm-up stretches is to prime the pump. Utilize all major muscle groups in a relatively slow, methodical build-up of intensity to be ready to rock and roll!

RI - Rest Interval refers to the recovery segment of the workout.

Track Workout/Speed Workout - My definition implies that you are working at 100% VO2 Max or higher. These workouts are rarely meant **to** be talking sessions. This doesn't mean that people don't congregate on the track to do less intense workouts but it does mean that unless I have specifically defined something else, your workout is at maximum effort for completing the given task.

VO2 Max - My definition is from USATF training. Use an all-out timed 2 mile run as a measurement for heart rate. Let's say you have finished your run and your 60 second pulse is 180. This is the measurement this book uses for VO2 Max.

Pacing - This is such an important part of improvement and is not well understood. People often get confused as to how to extrapolate different paces from one race.

For example, let's say you ran a half marathon in just under 2 hours. Good job! By taking this race time, we can extrapolate that you should be able to run 2 miles in about 16 minutes and a 10K in about 54 minutes. Why? Statistics show that other people who run certain distances in certain times often run new distances in related times.

Thus, our 2 hour half marathoner did just a tad over 9 minute miles for 13.1 miles. That same person will statistically run a 10K in a little under 54 minutes or about 8'45" per mile. Same person is expected to run 2 miles in about 16 minutes or 8 minute miles. This statistical person keeps running the shorter distances faster because there are fewer miles to cover. A marathon? The same person is expected to do about 4 hours 11 minutes or something around 9'30"/mile.

If you need a pace chart please like my page at www.facebook.com/gowowteam. Post a current race time, distance and the next race you want to train for (between 2 miles and 26.2). I will post your per lap pace time.

5K Pace - If you are already a racer you might have tried a 5K Race. Use this time for your calculation. Your pace will be your lap time over the duration of 3.1 miles.

10K Pace - Same story. Use your race time divided by 6.2 miles to get a current 10K time per mile. Then divide your mile time into 4 laps. Voila! 10K pace for workouts.

Warm-up by Jogging Easy or Walking - This segment of the workout is to be done at an easy pace in order to get the muscles moving gradually and allows you to avoid injury when you do the intense part that follows. 10 – 20 minutes total warm-up times include the jog or walk and the dynamic stretches. You want to feel that you are loose and warm, and ready to give the hard part of your session a body that is prepared for the challenge ahead.

Suggested Dynamic Warm-up Exercises (do some or all)
- Jumping Jacks
- Squats
- Upright bicycles – knee to opposite elbow
- Skaters in place
- Butt Kicks
- High Knees
- Karaoke's (crossovers)
- Striders
- Leg Swings

Track and Speed Workouts

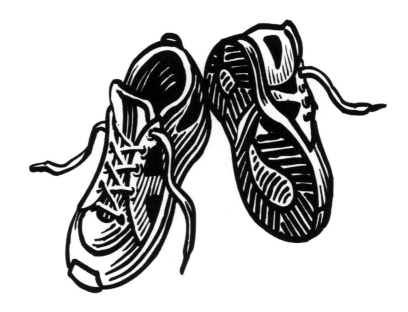

"If it's stupid, but it works, it's not stupid." - *Chinese proverb*

Run Faster Workout 1

Moderately Hard

- 800 meter warm-up plus dynamic stretches
- 1X800m with 1 lap walking/jogging recovery X 6 (at your 10K race pace)
- 2 laps jogging cool-down
- Stretch

Purpose: This is a good early-season workout if you have a decent base, and can handle continuous movement. It's a tougher workout than resting between sets. Be sure to try to do you hard laps at a 10K pace or faster. The goal is to be consistent throughout all 6 sets and pace your recovery laps to allow consistent effort on the hard laps.

Today's date _____

Amount of time for total workout _____

Your personal goals for this work out:

Comments:

"In the province of the mind, what one believes to be true either is true or becomes true." - John Lilly

Run Faster Workout 2

Least Hard

- 400 - 800 meter walk/run warm-up (depending on your speed) plus dynamic stretches
- 1 X 400m hard (running as much as possible) with 1 X 400 walking or walk/run for recovery, as needed. Repeat 6 times
- 2 laps walking or running cool-down
- Stretch

Purpose: A run/walk is a great way to get stronger and still do a track workout without intimidation. I highly recommend ordering a Gymboss. We at the WOW Team use these things all the time. They are inexpensive, easy to learn to use, and very helpful in getting faster incrementally. The link is http://interneka.com/affiliate/AIDLink.php?BID=14329&AID=39339

Today's date _____

Amount of time for total workout _____

Your personal goals for this work out:

Comments:

"Expecting the world to treat you fairly because you are a good person is a little like expecting the bull not to attack you because you are a vegetarian." - Dennis Wholey

Run Faster Workout 3

Least Hard

- 400 meter warm-up walking plus dynamic stretches
- Walk HARD for 1/2 lap, Easy 1/2 lap, Steady 1 lap
- Repeat 3-4 times
- Stretch

Purpose: Walking is possible for almost everyone. Early in the season or as a check on form, try to stay on the track lane line to see if you can keep your feet going straight ahead rather than side to side. This will make you a more efficient walker and keep you from certain injuries related to foot placement and balance.

Today's date _____

Amount of time for total workout _____

Your personal goals for this work out:

Comments:

"Baseball is 90 percent mental, and the other half is physical." - Yogi Berra

Run Faster Workout 4

Hardest

- 1 mile warm-up jog
- 400m at 5K pace, RI 1'30"
- 800m at 5K pace, RI 1'30"
- 1200m at 5K pace, RI 1'30"
- 1600m at 5K pace, RI 1'30"
- 1200m at 5K pace, RI 1'30"
- 800m at 5K pace, RI 1'30"
- 400m at 5K pace
- Cool down run 2 -4 laps
- Stretch

Purpose: Track Pyramid workouts test pacing and overall speed endurance. There will be a time when your legs will feel quite heavy. As you continue the workout, your body is adjusting, and for most of us the feeling abates and we can finish the workout strong.

Today's date _____

Amount of time for total workout _____

Your personal goals for this work out:

Comments:

"Everyone must row with the oars he has." - English Proverb

Run Faster Workout 5

Moderately Hard Group Run, run/walk, or walk

- 10 minutes warm-up to include 6 minutes on track and 4 minutes dynamic stretches
- Do 20 minutes at a hard pace (this can vary significantly and can include run/walk or walking)
- Return to starting line via shortest distance (may be turning around or crossing the field) and
- wait until everyone in the group is back.
- When you reach the finish line, STOP. You want to push yourself and pace yourself because you are not finished with the workout yet
- Rest 2 minutes once all are back
- Repeat entire set for another 20 minutes
- Cool-down jog or walk 1 - 2 laps
- Stretch

Purpose: Groups benefit from working out together, but the various paces can be challenging. By using times instead of distance, everyone can get a good workout with this design. If you have a coach or timer they can even whistle or yell when twenty minutes is up.

Today's date _____

Amount of time for total workout _____

Your personal goals for this work out:

Comments:

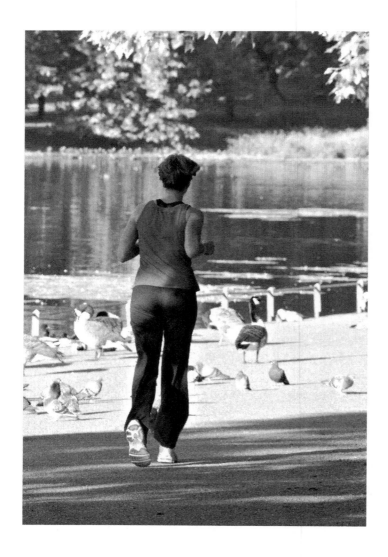

"All blame is a waste of time. No matter how much fault you find with another, and regardless of how much blame you place, it will not change you. The only thing blame does is keep the focus off you when you are looking for external reasons to explain your unhappiness or frustration. You may succeed in making another feel guilty of something, but you won't succeed in changing whatever it is about you that is making you unhappy." - Dr. Wayne Dyer

Run Faster Workout 6

Moderately Hard

- 10 min warm-up includes dynamic stretches
- 2 miles at Half Marathon Pace
- 3 min RI
- 1X1600m at 10K pace or faster
- 1 – 2 laps cool-down
- Stretch

Purpose: Pacing is essential for improvement and racing at different distances. This workout allows you to test a relatively steady half marathon pace (but remember this is your tentative race pace) and then adds a tougher mile to increase the intensity for a limited distance. This, in theory, may be how you want to run the last 3 miles of your actual race.

Today's date _____

Amount of time for total workout _____

Your personal goals for this work out:

Comments:

"Every adversity carries with it the seed of an equal or greater benefit." -
Napoleon Hill

Run Faster Workout 7

Hardest

- 10 minute warm-up, or more including dynamic stretches
- 10 striders
- Timed mile for 4 laps as hard as you can
- Rest 4 minutes (easy walking will help clear lactic acid)
- Do 2 miles at your half marathon pace
- 1-2 laps cool-down
- Stretching

Don't forget to bring a digital watch to time yourself. This really helps you stay on target even if you're not trying for a specific time goal.

Today's date _____

Amount of time for total workout _____

Your personal goals for this work out:

Comments:

*"One can never consent to creep when one feels an impulse to soar." -
Helen Keller*

Run Faster Workout 8

Hardest

- Warm-up 10 - 20 minutes
- 3 X (2 X 1200m) at 2 mile pace or faster
- 2 min RI between 1200's
- 4 minutes rest between sets
- Cool-down 10 minutes
- Stretch

Purpose: 1200's are difficult because they take focus, and a fair amount of fitness, to do them well. Test your pace on the first lap to determine if you can finish the workout at the intensity you have set. Walk, if feasible for the 2 minute break to recover from the lactic acid build-up.

Today's date _____

Amount of time for total workout _____

Your personal goals for this work out:

Comments:

"I believe that anyone can conquer fear by doing the things he fears to do, provided he keeps doing them until he gets a record of successful experiences behind him." - Eleanor Roosevelt

Run Faster Workout 9

Moderately Hard for Run, Walk, Run/Walk

- Warm-up 10 - 20 minutes
- 3 X (2 X 800m) at 5K pace or faster
- 2 minutes rest between 800's
- 4 minute rest between each set
- Cool-down 1 - 2 laps easy
- Stretch

Purpose: This workout is far enough that you can do it as a walking, run/walk, or even running workout. It is moderately hard because it gives you quite a bit of static rest in-between sets.

Today's date _____

Amount of time for total workout _____

Your personal goals for this work out:

Comments:

"I am not what I think. I am thinking what I think." - Eric Butterworth

Run Faster Workout 10

Least Hard Veg out Track Workout

- Set the music and earphones in 1 ear please, and stay in the outside lane
- Just keep moving to clear the cobwebs and ease the stress of life
- Stick with it for 30 minutes or more

Purpose: Everybody has down days, but often times the best recovery is to get out there and move!

Today's date _____

Amount of time for total workout _____

Your personal goals for this work out:

Comments:

"Dream what you dare to dream. Be where you want to go. Be what you want to be. Live!" – Richard Bach

Run Faster Workout 11

Hardest

- Standard warm-up
- 4 X 1600 with 400m RI (10K pace or faster)
- Cool down one or two laps
- Stretch

Purpose: This is a good workout for a half or full marathon training program, since it works at a pace faster than planned race pace. It should be done a bit further into the season since it requires stamina as well as speed.

Today's date _____

Amount of time for total workout _____

Your personal goals for this work out:

Comments:

"A difference, to be a difference, must make a difference." - Dr. James Farr

Run Faster Workout 12

Least Hard - Gymboss Track Workout for Walkers or Runners

- Beat the Clock! Bring your Gymboss for a run/walk session
- Standard warm-up
- Set your Gymboss for 8 minutes
- See how far you can get in 8 minutes. Run, walk, or vary it. Try to be constant with your breathing and listen to it as you move. For example run the straights, walk the curves or run 3/4 of the track, walk 1/4.
- After 8 minutes' walk, note where you finished and walk back to the start
- Repeat the exercise once or twice more trying to beat the distance you covered each time
- Cool down with 1 lap walk or jog
- Stretch

Purpose - Dual: This workout can be hard or easy depending on how you do it! Use it as an easy workout if you want to rest a bit, but put in some time. Use it as a tough workout by running hard each 8 minute set and try to cover more territory each time.

Today's date _____

Amount of time for total workout _____

Your personal goals for this work out:

Comments:

"A man without a plan for the day is lost before he starts." - Lewis K. Bendele

Run Faster Workout 13

Hardest

- 1 mile easy warm-up (5 – 10 minutes) plus dynamic stretching
- 1X800m with 1 lap jogging recovery X 8 (at your 5K race pace or faster)
- 2 laps jogging cool-down
- Stretch

Purpose: This is a good mid-season workout when you have a decent base and can handle continuous movement. It's a tougher workout than resting between sets. Be sure to try to do your hard laps at a 5K pace or faster. The goal is to be consistent throughout all the sets and pace your recovery laps to allow consistent effort on the hard laps.

Today's date _____

Amount of time for total workout _____

Your personal goals for this work out:

Comments:

"One dreamed of becoming somebody. Another remained awake and became." - Anonymous

Run Faster Workout 14

Moderately Hard

- 10 – 20 minute warm-up with dynamic stretching
- 2 X (4 X 400) at 10K pace or faster (faster is more difficult, of course), 1:30 RI
- 2:30 rest in between sets
- 10 minute cool-down
- Stretch

Purpose: You can modify the difficulty by adjusting the lap pace you run. Try to stay consistent throughout the workout, although I always like to run my last lap all out. That's just me, but it also helps with that final sprint push that tests everything you have, and might make the difference in how you place in a race.

Today's date _____

Amount of time for total workout _____

Your personal goals for this work out:

Comments:

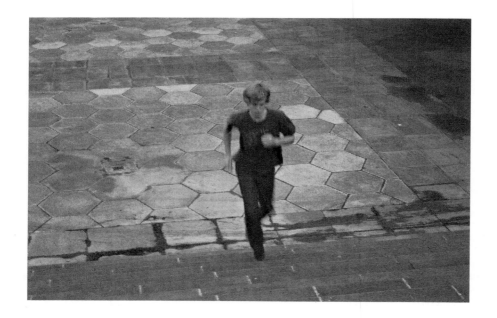

"Live out of your imagination instead of out of your memory." - Les Brown

Run Faster Workout 15

Hardest

- Non Track Location Gymboss practice - 2X2
- Use a land route that is approximately 3 miles to practice with your Gymboss. Set the
- increments for 2:2 (2 minutes and 2 minutes)
- Warm-up by walking or easy jogging for 5 minutes before starting you Gym Boss
- Start the Gymboss and run or walk as hard as you can for 2 minutes
- Take a walking break for two minutes. Keep moving but give yourself a pace that allows you to
- recover for the next hard segment
- Repeat hard/easy until you finish the course
- Cool down by walking 5 minutes and stretch

Purpose: This workout is truly a tempo or fartlek-type run. By using the Gymboss you really have to set stringent time segments for hard and easy parts of the workout. It takes having to look at your watch out of the equation. It also gives you regular breaks on a sustained distance. All of these pieces together will help you become a stronger athlete if you apply yourself. The work put in is definitely related to the gain at the other end.

Today's date _____

Amount of time for total workout _____

Your personal goals for this work out:

Comments:

"Never look down on anybody unless you're helping him up." - Jesse Jackson

Run Faster Workout 16

Least Hard

- Veg. out - De-stress - walk or jog for 30 minutes or more
- Keep a steady pace and listen to your breathing. Is it rhythmic? Does it guide your legs and set the pace for the workout? It should.
- At this low stress, easy pace you are making yourself do something when, otherwise you might skip the workout.

Purpose: To de-stress and appreciate the gift of movement, even on a tough day, is a wonderful bonus in life. Celebrate what is good, even when the bleakness pervades.

Today's date _____

Amount of time for total workout _____

Your personal goals for this work out:

Comments:

"It's important; but it's not serious." - Michael E. Angier

Run Faster Workout 17

Moderately Hard

- Warm-up 1 mile, easy followed by dynamic stretches
- 1 X 800m at 10K pace w/ 400m slow recovery jog – RI
- Repeat 4 – 6 times
- Cool down a full mile easy jogging or walking
- Stretch

Purpose: Because of the pace here, (10K) this workout is more designed for early season track or marathon distance races. A 10K pace on the track is relatively slow. Don't overdo the recovery lap by walking unless you are, in fact, a walker. In other words, give yourself time to recover but don't be lazy about it. We're working on your ability to sustain the hard segment without total recovery in between.

Today's date _____

Amount of time for total workout _____

Your personal goals for this work out:

Comments:

"Opportunities are usually disguised as hard work, so most people don't recognize them." - Ann Landers

Run Faster Workout 18

Moderately Hard

- Warm-up 1 - 2 miles, easy followed by dynamic stretches
- 1 X 1600m at 10K pace
- ½ mile RI easy continuous movement
- Repeat 3 times
- Cool down a full mile easy jogging or walking
- Stretch

Purpose: This continues the longer distance speed training, like the one above with a moderate pace of 10K. This workout is especially recommended for marathon distances and above.

Today's date _____

Amount of time for total workout _____

Your personal goals for this work out:

Comments:

"Dream lofty dreams, and as you dream, so shall you become. Your vision is the promise of what you shall one day be; your ideal is the prophecy of what you shall at last unveil." - James Allen

Run Faster Workout 19

Hardest

- Warm-up 1 mile, easy followed by dynamic stretches
- Run 400m at 5K pace
- 200m jog/walk recovery
- Run 800m at 5K pace
- 200m jog/walk recovery
- Run 1200m at 5K pace
- 200m jog/walk recovery
- Run 800m at 5K pace
- 200m jog/walk recovery
- Run 400m best effort (at your all out)
- Cool down walk or jog ½ mile
- Stretch

Purpose: Do this work out when you are well into your season. It is tough but it makes you feel great to do it. It's not too long, but every piece is taxing, including the short walk/jog segment in-between the hard "ladder" (also called a pyramid).

Today's date _____

Amount of time for total workout _____

Your personal goals for this work out:

Comments:

"Problems call forth our courage and our wisdom; indeed they create our courage and wisdom. It is only because of problems that we grow. It is for this reason that wise people learn not to dread but actually welcome problems." - M. Scott Peck

Run Faster Workout 20

Hardest

- Warm-up 1 mile, easy followed by dynamic stretches
- Run 400m at 5K pace
- 200m jog/walk recovery
- Run 800m at 5K pace
- 200m jog/walk recovery
- Run 1600m at 5K pace
- 200m jog/walk recovery
- Run 800m at 5K pace
- 200m jog/walk recovery
- Run 400m best effort (all out)
- Cool down walk or jog ½ mile, Stretch

Purpose: Variation on a theme. This workout and the one above it are pretty similar. However, I have learned that it is fun to have different workouts rather than same old, same old. Clearly running a mile takes more time than running 1200m. Either of them adds the element of good, solid pacing, along with the ability to endure the whole workout at a fast pace. Want to make it even harder? Change the pace to a 2 mile race pace!

Today's date _____

Amount of time for total workout _____

Your personal goals for this work out:

Comments:

"It's not the will to win, but the will to prepare to win that makes the difference." - Coach Bryant

Run Faster Workout 21

Moderately Hard

- 10-20 min warm up
- 1200m at 10K pace
- 1000m at 10K pace
- 800m at 10K pace
- 600m at 2 mile race pace
- 400m at 2 mile race pace
- 200m at all out pace
- All with 200m RI active recovery
- 10 min cool down
- Stretch

Purpose: Keep things interesting, vary the pace. It keeps getting harder speed-wise but shorter distance-wise. Variety is good.

Today's date _____

Amount of time for total workout _____

Your personal goals for this work out:

Comments:

"Forget mistakes. Forget failures. Forget everything except what you're going to do now, and do it. Today is your lucky day." - Will Durant

Run Faster Workout 22

Least Hard

- 10 - 20 min warm up
- 6 x 100 meter striders
- 100 meter recovery in-between
- 10 min cool down
- Stretch

Purpose: This is a good beginner's workout. Total time moving is 30 minutes plus striders to start getting your body used to moving hard without over-doing it. Striders should focus on good form: rhythmic breathing, mid-foot strike, quick foot lift and turnover and arms pulling.

Today's date _____

Amount of time for total workout _____

Your personal goals for this work out:

Comments:

"Forget mistakes. Forget failures. Forget everything except what you're going to do now, and do it. Today is your lucky day." - Will Durant

Run Faster Workout 23

Least Hard (first in set)

- 10-20 min easy warm up jog or walk with dynamic stretches
- 2 laps on track easy pace, focusing on rhythmic breathing, forceful out, deep chest intake
- 1 min rest
- 2 laps of track, faster pace, focusing on breathing, noticing the rhythm
- 1 min rest
- 2 laps on track, fastest pace possible to complete the set, focusing on breathing. All 3 sets should have similar rhythm for breathing. The difference will come from the power in your legs and arms and how much effort you can exert
- 2 laps easy walk or jog
- Stretch

Purpose: Breathing is the essential factor for most exercise. We are very limited in how long we can work without oxygen (anaerobically). By listening to and understanding our breathing rhythm, we can control our level of effort and thus how long we can work out.

Today's date _____

Amount of time for total workout _____

Your personal goals for this work out:

Comments:

"The fresh start is always an illusion but a necessary one." - Eleanor Clark

Run Faster Workout 24

Least Hard (second in set)

- 10-20 min easy warm up jog or walk with dynamic stretches
- 2 laps on track easy pace focusing on mid-foot landing, easy pace, foot touches down under or slightly behind body
- 1 min rest
- 2 laps of track, faster pace, focusing on mid-foot landing. Breathing stays steady, deep, and
- rhythmic
- 1 min rest
- 2 laps on track, fastest pace possible to complete the set, focusing on legs. All 3 sets should have similar rhythm for breathing. The difference will come from the power in your legs and arms and how much effort you can exert.
- 2 laps easy walk or jog
- Stretch

Purpose: Without legs, you are not able to run or walk. Almost everyone can walk, many can run, few can go fast. Why? Practice and repetition. This exercise trains your body to get stronger while using techniques that teach rhythm, power, and eventually, speed.

Today's date _____

Amount of time for total workout _____

Your personal goals for this work out:

Comments:

*"No man is lonely while eating spaghetti. It requires so much attention." -
Christopher Morley*

Run Faster Workout 25

Least Hard (third in set)

- 10-20 min easy warm up jog or walk with dynamic stretches
- 2 laps on track easy pace focusing on arms pulling straight back, elbows bent, for emphasis try to rub elbows on hips, bring fingers to hips. Fingers held loosely; do not extend forward above chest height
- 1 min rest
- 2 laps of track, faster pace, focusing on arms, utilize mid-foot landing. Breathing stays steady, deep, and rhythmic
- 1 min rest
- 2 laps on track, fastest pace possible to complete the set, focusing on arms. All 3 sets should have similar rhythm for breathing and good, mid-foot strike. The difference in power will come from the legs and arms and how much effort you can exert.
- 2 laps easy walk or jog
- Stretch

Purpose: With arms, legs, and breathing technique understood, YOU CONTROL the workout. To improve, you tweak one piece at a time, depending on your current goal.

Today's date _____

Amount of time for total workout _____

Your personal goals for this work out:

Comments:

Running Question?
How many days per week should you be doing strength training?

Answer: Strength training for distance runners should happen on a regular basis, maybe 2 - 3 times a week depending on the intensity and duration of the workout. Be sure to include upper and lower body exercises. Core exercise is a part of this, of course.

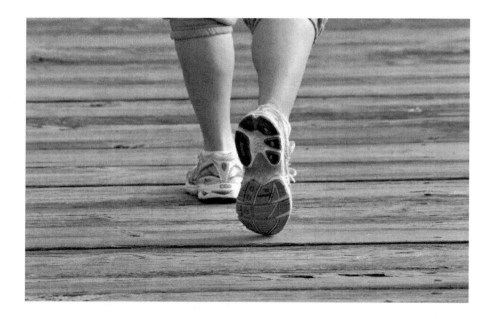

"I do get scared about the physical danger from drug dealers. But it's not in the same league as the danger I feel eating an $80 lunch with my privileged friends to discuss hunger and poverty. That's when my soul feels."- Kozol

Run Faster Workout 26

Least Hard to Moderately Hard

- 10-20 min easy warm up jog or walk with dynamic stretches
- 2 X 800m at goal race pace
- Jog easy between each 800
- 2 X 400m at goal pace
- 1 mile easy jogging cool down
- Stretch

Purpose: This workout is a good taper type workout, no matter what your race distance. Warm-up and cool down help get you in a comfortable mental state and the workout itself is an aid to reassure proper race pacing without over-doing the distance.

Today's date _____

Amount of time for total workout _____

Your personal goals for this work out:

Comments:

*"Action to be effective must be directed to clearly conceived ends." -
Jawaharlal Nehru*

Run Faster Workout 27

Least Hard to Moderately Hard

- 10-20 min easy warm up jog or walk with dynamic stretches
- 3 X 800m at goal race pace
- Jog easy between each 800
- 2 X 400m at goal pace
- 1 mile easy jogging cool down
- Stretch

Purpose: You set the pace based on your next race goal. Thus, if you plan to run a marathon at 10 min per mile your goal pace per lap would be 2'30". If you plan to run a 5K in 18'36, your lap pace would be 1'39" so this could be a relatively easy or moderately hard work out.

Today's date _____

Amount of time for total workout _____

Your personal goals for this work out:

Comments:

"Do not refuse a wing to the person who gave you the whole chicken." -
R.G.H. Siu

Run Faster Workout 28

Moderately Hard

- Warm up on track 5 – 10 min
- Upright Bicycle, knee to elbow, 10 on each side
- Butt Kicks, 20
- Speed Skate (in place) 20
- Hurdle forward and backward 10 in each direction, both legs
- Wall sit 12", dorsi-flex feet, 60 seconds
- Skip to end of straight, walk back with fast arms
- Repeat all 1 – 2 more times with final set doing exercises to fatigue
- Run 1 mile at 10K pace
- Cool down easy 2 laps
- Stretch

Purpose: This exercise works on technique and increasing strength and flexibility in the large muscle sets that is essential to staying injury free. The non-running exercises should be done relatively quickly but with full range of motion and control up and down, out and in. Do not bounce!

Today's date _____

Amount of time for total workout _____

Your personal goals for this work out:

Comments:

47

"Great occasions do not make heroes or cowards; they simply unveil them to the eyes. Silently and imperceptibly, as we wake or sleep, we grow strong or we grow weak, and at last some crisis shows us what we have become." - Bishop Westcott

Run Faster Workout 29

Hardest – Pyramid

- Warm up 1 mile plus dynamic stretches 5 – 10 min
- 1 X 400m at 2 mile pace. Rest 1 ½ minutes
- 1 X 800m at 2 mile pace. Rest 1 ½ minutes
- 1 X 1200m at 2 mile pace. Rest 1 ½ minutes
- 1 X 1 mile at 2 mile pace. Rest 1 ½ minutes
- 1 X 800m at 2 mile pace. Rest 1 ½ minutes
- 1 X 400m best pace and try to be fastest lap of all
- Cool down walk or jog 1-2 laps, Stretch

Purpose: Work these muscles hard at relatively short distances if you're an endurance runner, but pace yourself to finish the entire workout and save a bit of energy for the final lap. This workout finish may help you win your race or, at least gain some position by having a "kick" at the very end. This type of finish takes practice and mental preparation to stick with the pain just a bit longer.

Today's date _____

Amount of time for total workout _____

Your personal goals for this work out:

Comments:

"Do not wait; the time will never be just right. Start where you stand, and work with whatever tools you may have at your command, and better tools will be found as you go along." - Napoleon Hill

Run Faster Workout 30

Hardest - Just a bit harder than the previous pyramid

- Warm up 1 mile plus dynamic stretches 5 – 10 min
- 1 X 400m at 2 mile pace
- Jog or run easy 1 lap for recovery
- 1 X 800m at 2 mile pace
- Jog or run easy 1 lap for recovery
- 1 X 1200m at 2 mile pace
- Jog or run easy 1 lap for recovery
- 1 X 1 mile at 2 mile pace
- Jog or run easy 1 lap for recovery
- 1 X 800m at 2 mile pace
- Jog or run easy 1 lap for recovery
- 1 X 400m best pace and try to be fastest lap of all
- Cool down walk or jog 1-2 laps, Stretch

Purpose: Working with lactic acid is a skill, and the best athletes are better at it than most of us. When you get that heavy, burning feeling in your legs, lactic acid is building up in your system. Mental and physical practice can help us become more efficient and more accustomed to this discomfort. This exercise is all about working through that mental and physical pain.

Today's date _____

Amount of time for total workout _____

Your personal goals for this work out:
Comments:

"A narrow mind and a wide mouth usually go together." - Anonymous

Run Faster Workout 31

Hardest – Hill Workout

- Warm up 10 minutes easy jogging plus dynamic stretches 5 – 10 min
- Find a hill of moderate steepness. Ideally, it will have an easy way to get back down that is not as steep. However, you can walk down the same hill for your recovery.
- Run hard 1 – 2 minutes from the base to a point that you mark (or the crest of the hill)
- Recover by walking down or jogging easy around if you can make a circuit, allow 3 minutes
- Repeat for 30 – 45 minutes. Yikes! This should be about 6 - 9 sets
- Move easy, jog on the flats if possible for cool down
- Stretch

Purpose: You are topping out here with maximum effort and anaerobic impact. This will give you strength of form and mental focus in this peak workout effort. Not for the novice runner. Be well into your training when you do this.

Today's date _____

Amount of time for total workout _____

Your personal goals for this work out:

Comments:

"Repeat anything often enough and it will start to become you." - Tom Hopkins

Run Faster Workout 32

Moderately Hard

- Warm up easy 5 – 10 min plus dynamic stretching
- 1 X 400 at 5K pace
- Active recovery with 1 lap jogging
- Repeat 8 – 10 times
- Cool down 2 laps jogging
- Stretch

Purpose: A good mid-season workout to test endurance and speed at a calculated pace.

Today's date _____

Amount of time for total workout _____

Your personal goals for this work out:

Comments:

"Necessity makes even the timid brave." - Sallust

Run Faster Workout 33

Least Hard – Fartlek

- 5 min easy warm up plus dynamic stretching
- 1/8 track maximum pace (approximately 15 seconds full out)
- Run the remainder of the track easy
- Repeat for 30 minutes
- 10 min easy jog cool down
- Stretch

Purpose: Practice speed with plenty of recovery time. This is a good way to stay focused on your form, get in a good workout, and put in continuous movement to build endurance.

Today's date _____

Amount of time for total workout _____

Your personal goals for this work out:

Comments:

"Joy is the feeling of grinning on the inside." - Dr. Melba Colgrove

Run Faster Workout 34

Moderately Hard (Gymboss useful)

- Warm up a mile at an easy pace
- Keep moving into dynamic stretches with 10 of each: jumping jacks, high knees, butt kicks,
- skaters
- Move directly into half marathon pace for 3 – 4 miles at half marathon pace
- Strive for evenly paced laps each and every lap from start to finish
- Cool down 1 – 2 laps
- Stretch

Purpose: Get into the rhythm of your half marathon pace and tweak it so that it's a tough pace, but doable over and over, lap after lap. This teaches your mind and body how to work together and repeats the process until it becomes understood at both ends, literally your head and your feet! You can extend this workout for up to 10 or more miles, just get in the zone and stay focused!

Today's date _____

Amount of time for total workout _____

Your personal goals for this work out:

Comments:

"I hope that while so many people are out smelling the flowers, someone is taking the time to plant some." - Herbert Rappaport

Run Faster Workout 35

Hardest

- Warm up a mile at an easy pace with dynamic stretching too
- 400m "ins and outs" - start out easy for half a lap
- Pick up pace to 10K speed for half a lap
- Repeat 5 times
- Pick up pace to 2 mile speed for half a lap, first half lap easy
- Repeat 5 times
- Run 400m at 2 mile pace
- Run 400m easy recovery lap
- Repeat 2 times
- Cool down 2 – 4 laps
- Stretch

Purpose: You are "upping the ante" while getting more fatigued. This workout takes mental confidence, stamina, and a "can-do" attitude. It is good to have a strong base because otherwise you are setting yourself up for injury.

Today's date _____

Amount of time for total workout _____

Your personal goals for this work out:

Comments:

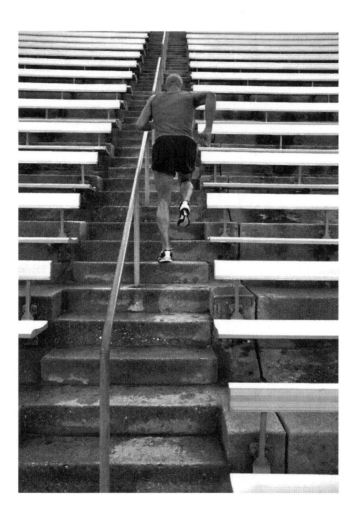

"The greatest of all mistakes is to do nothing because you can only do a little. Do what you can." - Sydney Smith

Run Faster Workout 36

Moderately Hard

- More fartlek
- Start with easy running for 5 – 10 minutes
- Move directly into the fartlek workout
- Run the straights moderately hard and the curves for recovery (you can also do this with city blocks or other incremental landmarks)
- Keep it up for 20 – 50 min
- Easy laps for total workout to equal 60 min
- Stretch

Purpose: Fartlek lets you work on speed and endurance. The difficult part is to keep pushing yourself for the duration of the workout. Novice runners can do limited speed sets while more experienced runners should do most of the workout with a reasonable amount of intensity (aka pain). By pain, I mean hard fast segments with max speed. If you actually feel pain somewhere, be careful because muscles usually hurt afterwards, not during the workout. If you feel the "burn" in your muscles, that is usually good. If you feel other kind of pain it may be a sign to pull back. *"Better safe than sorry."*

Today's date _____

Amount of time for total workout _____

Your personal goals for this work out:

Comments:

"It ain't over 'til it's over." - Yogi Berra

Run Faster Workout 37

Least Hard

- Warm-up to include 2 laps on track
- Add 5 min dynamic warm-up
- Skip the straights; jog the curves, 1 lap
- Side step the straights, jog the curves, 1 lap
- Striders on the straights, jog the curves, 1 lap
- Arms pulling steady and powerful on the straights, easy jog the curves
- 2 miles continuous, focusing on form. Talking OK. This is a low intensity workout.
- Stretch

Purpose: It seems than many of us have trouble with side movements, power bursts (like skipping and striders) and utilizing our arms. This workout focuses on these shortcomings and also gives us time to build up steady mileage as a base to keep us from getting injured.

Today's date _____

Amount of time for total workout _____

Your personal goals for this work out:

Comments:

"Be smart, be intelligent and be informed." - Tony Allasandra

Run Faster Workout 38

Moderately Hard Tempo Run

- 2 miles warm up talking
- 3 miles tempo, not able to talk more than a few words at a time. For more accuracy use your half marathon or 10K pace
- 1 mile cool down
- Stretch

Purpose: A 6 mile workout with 3 miles at a good clip is a good workout early in the season when you already have a base. This distance is excellent for mid-week workouts. Just change up the amount of miles you do at the harder pace as the season goes on.

Today's date _____

Amount of time for total workout _____

Your personal goals for this work out:

Comments:

"Having once decided to achieve a certain task, achieve it at all costs of tedium and distaste. The gain in self-confidence of having accomplished a tiresome labor is immense." - Thomas Arnold Bennett

Run Faster Workout 39

Moderately Hard to Most Difficult

- Warm-up 10 - 20 minutes plus get in some dynamic stretches
- Run 1000m, 2000m, 1000m, 1000m at 5K (more difficult) or 10K pace
- All with 400m recovery lap in-between
- Note: you will be running/jogging during the recovery phase as well as the hard phase.
- Cool-down 10 minutes
- Stretch

Purpose: This workout uses a different distance than normal, which changes things up in your brain as well as your body. While it is good to teach the body certain paces and patterns; it is also beneficial to put in something unusual once in a while for both muscular and mental/neurological benefit.

Today's date _____

Amount of time for total workout _____

Your personal goals for this work out:

Comments:

"It is too easy to give up on ourselves when we let who we are today prevent us from seeing what we can be tomorrow." - Michael Josephson

Run Faster Workout 40

Hardest

- Warm-up 1 mile easy
- 5 -10 min dynamic stretches including striders
- Continuous: 400s: 400m fast, 400m RI with fast laps at 2 mile pace or faster
- RI lap be sure to jog it, no walking, you will still be fatigued when you start the next hard lap
- 40 - 50 minutes total hard segment
- 2 laps walk or jog
- Stretch

Purpose: Getting used to the lactic acid build-up when your body cannot exchange energy bi-products and toxins fast enough is a way to adapt to a mind-body connection that allows you to keep going even when it is quite intense and uncomfortable.

Today's date _____

Amount of time for total workout _____

Your personal goals for this work out:

Comments:

"Happiness isn't an outside job, it's an inside job." - Anonymous

Run Faster Workout 41

Moderately Hard

- 10 – 20 minute warm-up to include jogging plus dynamic stretching
- 4 - 6 X 800m at 5K pace with 1:30 RI
- 10 minute cool-down to include walking or jogging and static stretching

Purpose: Good mid-season workout for building confidence. You should be able to do this # of sets without too much trouble if you have a decent base. You are giving yourself a static rest too.

Today's date _____

Amount of time for total workout _____

Your personal goals for this work out:

Comments:

"No problem can stand the assault of sustained thinking." – Voltaire

Run Faster Workout 42

Hardest

- Warm-up 10 - 20 minutes including dynamic stretching
- 800m at 5K or 2 mile pace
- 400m active recovery jog
- 1200m at same pace
- 400m active recovery jog
- 800m at same pace
- 400m active recovery jog
- Repeat above set one more time
- 400m all-out
- Cool-down 1 - 2 laps easy
- Stretch

Purpose: A tough workout to do when you are strong and well into your training season. This workout will test your endurance, show your mental focus, and give you a morale boost if you do it when you are capable of handling the challenge. Add some quick energy 15 min or so before you get started in the form of GU or some type of high carb, easily digested energy source. Or, at least have this on hand as this workout will take its toll on your energy systems!

Today's date _____

Amount of time for total workout _____

Your personal goals for this work out:

Comments:

"A heart to resolve, a head to contrive, and a hand to execute." - Edward Gibbon

Run Faster Workout 43

Hardest

- Warm-up 10 - 20 minutes including dynamic stretching
- Run a timed 2 mile to beat your former time. Pace yourself, don't go out too fast!
- Cool down 1 – 2 miles easy walk or jog
- Stretch

Purpose: See how much you've improved. Get in a good warm-up but don't feel drained when you start this workout. Feel ready, and full of energy. Get into the rhythm immediately and stick with it. Try the mantra "light legs lift". Stay in focus; monitor 1) breathing, 2) legs, 3) arms. 8 laps here we come!

Today's date _____

Amount of time for total workout _____

Your personal goals for this work out:

Comments:

Tip from Coach Stephanie: Bring a digital watch to time yourself. This really helps you stay on target even if you're not trying for a specific time goal. If you can't stay within a certain rhythm it may be a day to walk for peace of mind and skip the pressure workout.

Run Faster Workout 44

Hardest

- 10 – 20 min warm-up to include jogging plus dynamic stretching
- 2 X 4 X 400m (each as fast as you can do it and still finish the workout)
- 1:30 RI
- 2:30 rest in between sets
- 5 - 10 min cool down easy walk or jog
- Stretch

Purpose: All-out effort and pacing combined is what the elite racers have fine-tuned. When you work at this level, be rested and feel confident. Then, go like you mean it. Persevere. Remember, this is an endurance workout not a 100m sprinter's workout. The difference? The energy system you are fine tuning.

Today's date _____

Amount of time for total workout _____

Your Personal Goals for this work out:

Comments:

"Relentless, repetitive self-talk is what changes our self-image." - Denis E. Waitley

Run Faster Workout 45

Moderately Hard to Hardest

- Follow the leader. This is a good workout to do with other folks around
- Doing track workouts, in general, is so much easier with other folks around, right?
- Warm-up 10 - 20 minutes including jogging and dynamic stretching
- Line up with 2 - 4 runners directly behind each other. The slower runner should be at the front to start and, for best effect; runners have to be pretty close in pace. If you have a disparity with pacing it will make the workout hard for the slower paced runners and moderate for the faster runners. Still a good workout for all.
- Run 1 mile hard with 400m easy recovery lap or, if you have pace disparity, let the slower runners rest while the faster runners run a recovery lap
- Run 2 miles hard with 800m recovery laps
- Run 2X800m with 400m recovery lap after first set then go to
- Cool down 1 - 2 laps, Stretch

Purpose: Working with others is a great way to push ourselves. This exercise gets you directly involved with your peers. Think positively. Try it! If it's too hard, do part with the group and the rest on your own.

Today's date _____

Amount of time for total workout _____

Your personal goals for this work out:

Comments:

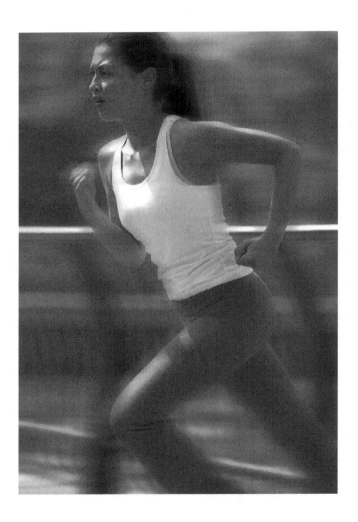

"Courage is not the absence of fear, but rather the judgment that something else is more important than fear." - Ambrose Bierce

Run Faster Workout 46

Least Hard

- Veg. out workout to de-stress
- Start from right where you are. No driving if possible.
- Head toward the most beautiful area you can reach in 30 minutes or less and walk or jog your way to some peace of mind and increased energy
- Total time 60 minutes
- Just do it

Purpose: We all have days when we need a physical and emotional boost. I have never had a day when I got out and did something that I felt worse afterward. NEVER!

Today's date _____

Amount of time for total workout _____

Your personal goals for this work out:

Comments:

"A truly creative person rids him or herself of all self-imposed limitations."
- Gerald G Jampolsky

Run Faster Workout 47

Hardest

- Warm-up easy 1 mile. Follow up with dynamic stretching.
- Finish warm-up with 4 sets of striders (20m, jog back)
- 8 X 200m all-out w/ a 200m recovery jog
- Cool-down 2 miles easy
- Stretch

Purpose: You are testing your mid-distance energy system here meaning the 100m to 800m almost anaerobic workout. For a good explanation that's not too detailed, here is a link
http://www.shapesense.com/fitness-exercise/articles/exercise-energy-systems.aspx#lacticanaerobic

Today's date _____

Amount of time for total workout _____

Your personal goals for this work out:

Comments:

"The error of youth is to believe that intelligence is a substitute for experience; while the error of age is to believe that experience is a substitute for intelligence." - Anonymous

Run Faster Workout 48

Least Hard, Even Easy

- When the world won't let you get off and you need a mental and physical break from where you right now, this is your workout
- Stand up, put on the walking or running shoes and head out the door. Don't get in the car if you can avoid it. Just start moving
- Walk (or jog) to the most beautiful spot you can reach in 30 minutes or less
- Keep walking for 60 minutes total
- Get lost in the wonder of the natural world and in the beauty of movement
- Forget the worries of the day
- When you finish you will be a different person

Purpose: Life or work getting to you? When things are so bleak or exhausting that hanging in there is doing more damage than good. Go for a walk or easy jog. I have never done this type of workout, under duress, when I didn't return feeling better. NEVER! Give yourself a break.

Today's date _____

Amount of time for total workout _____

Your personal goals for this work out:

Comments:

"Begin to be now what you will be hereafter." - Saint Jerome

Run Faster Workout 49

Hardest

- Warm-up easy 1 mile. Follow up with dynamic stretching.
- Finish warm-up with 4 sets of striders (20m, jog back)
- 2 X 200m all-out with a 200m jog recovery
- 2 X 400m all-out with a 200m jog recovery
- Rest 9 minutes, easy walking or static, stand in place, after you regain you composure from the
- first set
- Repeat set
- Cool-down jog 1 mile
- Stretch

Purpose: More development of the lactic acid anaerobic glycolytic energy cycle (100m – 800m, 7-10 secs – 90 seconds). Why would endurance runners do this? For the kick at the end of a race, and for fine tuning your running. It is well known that elite athletes can tolerate a high level of discomfort. This workout works at a high level of intensity and thus, discomfort.

Today's date _____

Amount of time for total workout _____

Your personal goals for this work out:

Comments:

"Bloom where you are planted." - Nancy Reader Campion (Aunt Grace)

Run Faster Workout 50

Moderately Hard

- Warm-up easy 1 mile. Follow up with dynamic stretching.
- Run 6 X 400m at your HMP or 10K pace
- Active RI of 400m in-between each lap
- Cool down jog 1 mile
- Stretch

Purpose: This is a good mid-season workout or a taper week run. Stay in the game by keeping up a track regimen but calm yourself with a workout that is very doable when you are well trained. And you are well trained and ready to kick _____ in your race!

Today's date _____

Amount of time for total workout _____

Your personal goals for this work out:

Comments:

"Imitation is a necessity of human nature." - Oliver Wendell Holmes, Jr.

Run Faster Workout 51

Hardest

- Warm-up easy 1 mile. Follow up with dynamic stretching.
- Finish warm-up with 4 sets of striders (20m, jog back)
- Run 1000m (2 ½ laps)
- Recover with a 400m jog
- Run 2000m
- Recover with a 400m jog
- Run 1000m
- Recover with a 400m jog
- Run 1000m
- Cool down 1 – 2 laps
- Stretch

Purpose: Pace yourself at 2 miles or 5K pace and you will be working hard! This is pushing your anaerobic threshold, which is great for endurance running. Be sure you have a good base and feel rested for this one.

Today's date _____

Amount of time for total workout _____

Your personal goals for this work out:

Comments:

"In the middle of every difficulty ,lies opportunity." - Albert Einstein

Run Faster Workout 52

Moderately Hard

- Reverse ladder starts at the top and comes down
- Warm-up easy 1 mile. Follow up with dynamic stretching.
- Run 1200m (3 laps) at 10K pace, 200m RI
- Run 1000m, 200m RI
- Run 800m, 200m RI
- Run 600m, 200m RI
- Run 400m, 200m RI
- Run 200m all-out
- Cool-down walk or jog 2 laps
- Stretch

Purpose: This workout will help you stay consistent with a pace, while changing the distance. Your 10K pace is not all-out by any means, but when you keep working at it from these shorter distances, you can train your mind and body to get used the feeling. Compute your lap times ahead of time and bring with you so you don't have to think about them while you run. Just check your notes.

Today's date _____

Amount of time for total workout _____

Your personal goals for this work out:

Comments:

"Exhilaration is that feeling you get just after a great idea hits you, and just before you realize what's wrong with it." - Rex Harrison

Run Faster Workout 53

Least Hard

- 10 minute walk/run warm-up plus dynamic stretches
- Do 1 mile hard without stopping, either run walk, walk, or run, whichever is your best effort. Try to pace each lap the same.
- Take a 2 lap recovery then repeat the whole set
- 2 laps jogging cool-down
- Stretch

Purpose: You are at a point where you want to practice what it feels like to be racing. Try it out. Do your best. Revel in your earned level of fitness! Go for it! You are ready for this.

Today's date _____

Amount of time for total workout _____

Your personal goals for this work out:

Comments:

"Nothing great was ever achieved without enthusiasm." - Ralph Waldo Emerson

Run Faster Workout 54

Hardest

- Warm up 1 mile easy plus dynamic stretches (jumping jacks, etc.)
- 3 - 5 X 1600 (10K pace or faster)
- 400m RI continuous movement, easy jogging or even walking
- 2 - 4 laps cool down jog
- Stretch

Purpose: Get that pace tucked smoothly into your body and mind, nice and neat and steady. This pace, if you keep a positive attitude might be a good goal for some future half marathon or 10 mile race.

Today's date _____

Amount of time for total workout _____

Your personal goals for this work out:

Comments:

"Any day above ground is a good day." - Anonymous

Run Faster Workout 55

Least Hard

- 10 minute walk/run warm-up plus dynamic stretches
- 1 X 400m hard (running as much as possible) with
- 1 X 400 walking or walk/run for recovery, as needed
- Repeat 6 times
- 2 laps walking or running cool-down
- Stretch

Purpose: Use your previous workouts to apply yourself to a hard, running, track workout. With walking for recovery, rather than standing, you still you have no time off. It's just a difference in pace. Try to finish the whole thing.

Today's date _____

Amount of time for total workout _____

Your personal goals for this work out:

Comments:

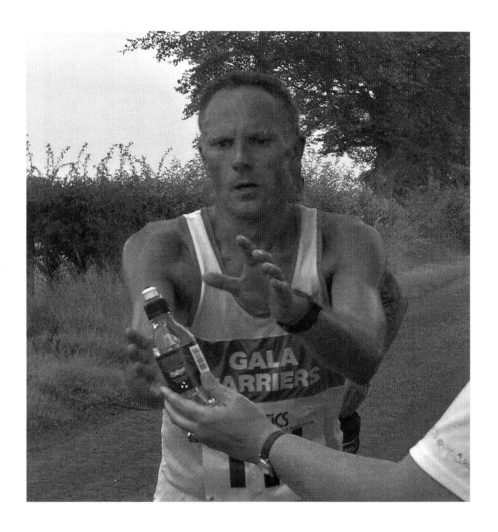

"Stupid questions are better than stupid mistakes." - Anonymous

Run Faster Workout 56

Hardest

- Warm-up 10 - 20 minutes to include dynamic stretches and jogging
- Add some striders just before doing the 100's
- 5 X 1000m with 400m RI at 2 mile pace
- 5 - 10 minute cool down, stretch

Purpose: When you have a good base, you want to push your pace and your distance at the same time. This is a distance runner's workout, not for beginners and not for sprinters.

Today's date _____

Amount of time for total workout _____

Your personal goals for this work out:

Comments:

"Things may come to those who wait, but only the things left by those who hustle." - Abraham Lincoln.

Run Faster Workout 57

Least Hard

- Warm-up 10 - 20 minutes
- Walk 400m hard with arms pumping, Rest 60 seconds or count of 60
- Do 30 pushups or to fatigue, whichever comes first
- Immediately turn on your side and do a side plank with arm lift to a count of 60 or fatigue, whichever comes first. Change sides and repeat.
- Lying on your back do tabletop circles with your legs to a count of 60
- Move to your side, resting on your elbows, and circle leg in a forward direction then reverse, each for a count of 30. Change sides and repeat.
- Run or walk a mile at a steady pace (4 laps)
- Repeat this circuit one more time
- Stretch

Purpose: Good workout for anyone injured, or ready for a strength and technique circuit workout

Today's date _____

Amount of time for total workout _____

Your personal goals for this work out:

Comments:

"Enthusiasm is contagious. Not having enthusiasm is also contagious." - *Anonymous*

Run Faster Workout 58

Hardest

Speed Track Workout for half marathoners
Assuming you are in a 12 week training program, Week 11 will often be your hardest workout. This holds true for 10K and half marathon races for most athletes.

- 10 minute warm-up plus dynamic stretches
- 1 X 800m hard, jog 1 lap
- 1 X 1200 hard, jog 1 lap
- 1 X 1600 hard, jog 1 lap,
- 1 X 2 miles hard
- 2 laps jogging cool-down
- Stretch

Purpose: Push hard; make an all-out training effort on your last, non-taper workout. If run/walkers choose to try this workout, they might not get all the way to the 2 miles due to time. All workouts are based on 60 minutes for the whole thing (including warm up and cool down.)

Today's date _____

Amount of time for total workout _____

Your personal goals for this work out:

Comments:

"In the final analysis, each of us is responsible for what we are. We cannot blame it on our mothers." - Helen Lawrenson

Run Faster Workout 59

Moderately Hard

- Warm-up 10 - 20 minutes to include dynamic stretches and jogging
- 1200 @ 10K pace with 2 minute rest
- 800 @ 10K pace with 2 minute rest
- 400 @ 10K pace with 2 minute rest
- 400 with lap time faster than any of the above laps
- 2 lap cool-down, Stretch

Purpose: Get that lactic acid rushing through you, so that your body gets a sense of what it all feels like and gets an opportunity to deal with it, too. A 10K pace is relatively slow on the track so focus on form and function - breathing, legs, and arms.

Today's date _____

Amount of time for total workout _____

Your personal goals for this work out:

Comments:

"Example has more followers than reason." - Bovee

Run Faster Workout 60

Least Hard

- 10 minute walk/run warm-up plus dynamic stretches
- Run or walk up stadium stairs staying on the balls of your feet, driving with your knees, power from arms and legs. Do this for approx. 5 minutes.
- Run an easy recovery lap on the track
- Do 20 squats, 10 - 20 pushups, 10 squat jumps, 50 table top crunches, 1 minute wall sit
- (Repeat entire sequence for a harder workout)
- 2 laps jogging cool-down
- Stretch

Purpose: Check your strength, overall body movement coordination, and stamina. When you do this work out fast, it takes all the abilities listed above. If you slow things down, you can focus on improving an area where you know you are weak (stairs for example and the stamina to complete 5 minutes of them).

Today's date _____

Amount of time for total workout _____

Your personal goals for this work out:

Comments:

Running Question?
How do you calculate your 10K pace? Answer on next page.

Answer: To calculate a 10K pace for track workouts you can use a prior, recent 10K race or set up a 10K (or 6 mile) course and time yourself running as fast as you can. Break that 10K time into minutes per mile. You can find charts online or use a calculator. Divide a mile by 4 and you will have a 10K lap time for the track.

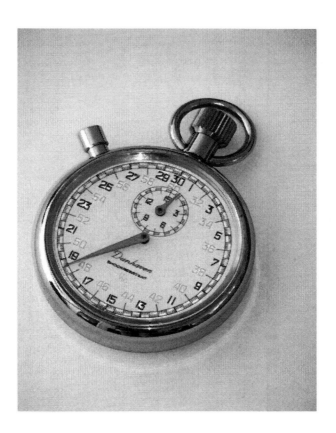

"Man who stand on hill with mouth open will wait long time for roast duck to drop in." - Confucius

Run Faster Workout 61

Moderately Hard

- Warm-up 10 - 20 minutes to include dynamic stretches and jogging
- 1600 @ 10K pace with 2 minute rest
- 1200 @ 10K pace with 2 minute rest
- 800 @ 10K pace with 2 minute rest
- 400 with lap time faster than any of the above laps
- 2 - 4 lap cool-down
- Stretch

Purpose: Ladders, like the one above are good for pacing. Try to keep your pace even until the final 400 at the end of the set. For a harder workout you could repeat the whole thing one more time.

Today's date _____

Amount of time for total workout _____

Your personal goals for this work out:

Comments:

"Behold the turtle: He only makes progress when he sticks his neck out." - James Bryant Conant

Run Faster Workout 62

Least Hard

Technique Track Workout

- Warm up 10 minutes of jogging or walking followed by 5 minutes of dynamic stretches
- Walk hard or run 1/2 lap
- Skip 1/2 lap
- Walk 1 lap to recover
- Sidestep 1/2 lap, swinging arms across the body to balance out the leg movement. Lead with right leg for the first half lap
- Reverse legs for next 1/2 lap, leading with left leg
- Walk 1 lap to recover
- Repeat with as much time as you have for the workout
- 5 minutes of easy walking or jogging for cool down
- Stretch

Purpose: For many novice runners and walkers, balance, stamina, coordination, and complimentary muscle groups really need to be worked on. This workout attempts to get your heart pumping by using different muscle sets and different moves than those specifically used for running and walking. This is an excellent workout for injury prevention.

Today's date _____

Amount of time for total workout _____

Your personal goals for this work out:

Comments:

"True happiness comes from the joy of deeds well done, the zest of creating things new." - Antoine de Saint-Exupery

Run Faster Workout 63

Moderately Hard

Track Taper Workout

- **5K Experienced Taper** - Do standard warm up
- Then run a 2 mile race pace run followed by 1 - 2 miles cool down and stretch
- Really focus on your pace and maintaining that hard, powerful level of breathing, legs, and arms that will take you through 3.1 miles on race day

- **5K First Timers -** Start with standard warm-up and dynamic stretches. Add 1 mile at your assumed race pace; recover with 1 lap of easy walking. Repeat this once more then finish with 1 -2 miles easy walk, run walk, or jogging, your choice. Stretch

Purpose: The purpose of both workouts listed is for you to perform at close to race pace but without the distance. Half marathoners generally taper for about a week, 5K is usually only a few days. This is why the 5K Intermediate Taper Workout is more sustained in the final week of training than for half marathoners.

Today's date _____

Amount of time for total workout _____

Your personal goals for this work out:

Comments:

"Wisdom is meaningless until our own experience has given it meaning." -
Bergen Evans

Run Faster Workout 64

Hardest

- Warm up 10 minutes of jogging or walking followed by 5 minutes of dynamic stretches
- 3 X (2X1200m with 2 min moving RI)
- 4 minutes rest between each set
- 5 minutes cool down
- Stretch

Purpose: Note the increase in distance. If you are not doing some type of cross training that addresses balance and other muscle sets, you may be better advised to try the "easier" workouts that are focused more on injury prevention. The "harder" workouts are geared to increased speed and neuromuscular adaptation at different, hard, distances.

Today's date _____

Amount of time for total workout _____

Your personal goals for this work out:

Comments:

"Not failure, but low aim is a sin." - Benjamin E. Mayes

Run Faster Workout 65

Least Hard

- Warm up 10 minutes of jogging or walking followed by 5 minutes of dynamic stretches
- Do 8 - 12 X 400m at 2 mile pace or faster (all out) with 2 minutes RI
- 1 - 2 laps easy cool down
- Stretch

Purpose: The aim is to gain a sense of speed, power, and discomfort. 400's start off feeling hard but get easier by the end of the workout because they are finished in only one lap! Sprinters may not agree but we are distance runners so 400m is pretty darn short!

Today's date _____

Amount of time for total workout _____

Your personal goals for this work out:

Comments:

"After all is said and done, more is said than done." - American proverb

Run Faster Workout 66

Moderately Hard

- 10 minute warm-up plus dynamic stretches
- 4 X 1 mile with 1 lap walking/jogging recovery (at your 10K race pace)
- 2 laps jogging cool-down
- Stretch

Purpose: 10K pace is not an all-out lap. If you can bump it up to 5K pace or even 2 mile pace that's great. Be sure to plan to finish the whole thing though. Strategy matters. This is a good mid-season workout when you have a decent base and can handle continuous movement. It's a tougher workout than resting between sets. Be sure to try to do your hard laps at a 10K pace or faster. The goal is to be consistent throughout all the sets and pace your recovery laps to allow consistent effort on the hard laps.

Today's date _____

Amount of time for total workout _____

Your personal goals for this work out:

Comments:

"Achieve success in any area of life by identifying the optimum strategies and repeating them until they become habits." - Karl Wilhelm von Humboldt

Run Faster Workout 67

Hardest

- 10 minute warm-up plus dynamic stretches
- 1 X 800m hard with 2 min active RI
- 1 X 1200 hard with 2 min active RI
- 1 X 1600 with 2 min active RI
- 1 X 1200 (same deal)
- 1 X 800 (same)
- 2 - 4 laps jogging cool-down
- Stretch

Purpose: Run hard, but try to pace yourself to finish the workout.

Today's date _____

Amount of time for total workout _____

Your personal goals for this work out:

Comments:

"Expecting the world to treat you fairly because you are a good person is a little like expecting the bull not to attack you because you are a vegetarian." - Dennis Wholey

Run Faster Workout 68

Moderately Hard

Injured, Base Building, and Strength Workout with Gymboss (set for 60 seconds and 30 second intervals)

- Warm-up 10 - 20 minutes
- Upright pushups for 60 seconds, 30 seconds break
- One leg, Lateral pull with resistance for 60 seconds, 30 seconds break
- Change legs, 30 second break
- Chest Press with resistance, split leg stance for 60 seconds
- 50 squats, 1 lap hard
- 50 zombie kicks, each side, 1 lap hard
- 50 leg swings, each side, 1 lap hard
- 50 calf raises, single leg, each side, 1 lap easy
- Repeat as far as you can get
- 5 - 10 minute cool down, stretch

Purpose: Often when runners are injured, it is because the opposing muscles, what they use when they run, are not strong enough. This workout includes some strengthening and some running, for a balance of both.

Today's date _____

Amount of time for total workout _____

Your personal goals for this work out:

Comments:

"Our energy is in proportion to the resistance it meets. We attempt nothing great but from a sense of the difficulties we have to encounter, we persevere in nothing great but from a pride in overcoming them." - William Hazlitt

Run Faster Workout 69

Hardest

- Warm up 1 mile easy plus dynamic stretches (jumping jacks, etc.)
- 2 X 1200 at 5K or 2 mile all out pace (3 laps) with 1 lap easy in-between
- 2 X 800 with 1 lap easy in-between (same pace as above)
- 1 X 400 all out, hard as you can go!
- Cool-down lap or two and stretch

Purpose: 4 + miles at a good clip is a real confidence booster and a tough workout

Today's date _____

Amount of time for total workout _____

Your personal goals for this work out:

Comments:

Running Question?
How do you determine your MAXIMUM Heart Rate? Answer on next page...

Answer: Your maximum heart rate can be determined by running 2 miles as fast as you are able then taking your pulse immediately following. Some people use other methods, too but this one is OK'd by US Track and Field and I like it.

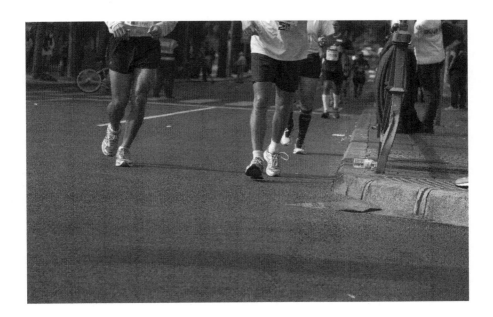

"Failures are divided into two classes-those who thought and never did, and those who did and never thought." - John Charles Salak

Run Faster Workout 70

Least Hard

- Warm up 10 minutes of jogging or walking followed by 5 minutes of dynamic stretches
- Walk hard or run continuously for 1 full lap, staying on the track lane line when landing. Rest 3 minutes
- Lap 2 - Listen to your breathing and make sure you have a rhythm to it - deep and steady. Move as fast as you can all the way around the track, aware and in control of your breathing. Rest 3 minutes
- Lap 3 - Focus on your legs and landing "light" (minimal heel strike with quick pickup of your legs) head around the track fast and focused. Rest 3 minutes
- Lap 4 - Pick up arms and PULL back as you run hard, breathing, with "light legs" and strong arms all the way around the track
- Rest 3 minutes
- Repeat with as much time as you have for the workout
- 5 minutes of easy walking or jogging for cool down. Stretch

Purpose: This uses balance, technique, and puts all the pieces together in a fast setting, but with the goal to improve your overall strength and technique. It helps you to start "listening" to your body. This is my "go to" workout and racing goal as I go through each piece: 1 - breathing (rhythmic and full), 2 - legs (light and strong), 3 - arms (pulling and powerful).

Today's date _____

Amount of time for total workout _____

Your personal goals for this work out:
Comments:

94

"It is easy to sit up and take notice. What is difficult is getting up and taking action." - Al Batt

Run Faster Workout 71

Moderately Hard

- Warm up 10 minutes of jogging or walking followed by 5 minutes of dynamic stretches
- Do 6 X 800m at 2 mile pace or faster (all out) with 90 seconds static RI
- 5 minutes cool down
- Stretch

Purpose: So much of running well is pacing. An 800m run is quite different than a 400m workout. You also are getting less rest time here. Keep the pace steady. Finish the workout by being conservative on your first lap and determining what it takes to complete the rest of it. Remember, you have 6 sets to complete.

Today's date _____

Amount of time for total workout _____

Your personal goals for this work out:

Comments:

"If you always do what you've always done, you'll always get what you've always got." Doug Kaufmann

Run Faster Workout 72

Hardest

Base Building and Strength Workout
- Warm-up 10 - 20 minutes to include dynamic stretches and jogging
- Striders for 50 yards X 3
- 10 pushups, 1 lap all out
- 20 squats, 1 lap all out
- 30 zombie kicks, 1 lap all out
- 40 leg swings, 1 lap all out
- 50 calf raises, 1 lap easy
- Repeat as far as you can get
- 5 - 10 minute cool down, stretch

Purpose: Cross training, strength training, and even just varying workouts makes your body happy. This can be done at different times during your training phases with more intensity as you get in better shape.

Today's date _____

Amount of time for total workout _____

Your personal goals for this work out:

Comments:

"Goals should be SMART: S = Specific; M = Measurable; A = Assignable (who does what); R =Realistic; T = Time related." - Anonymous

Run Faster Workout 73

Moderately Hard

- 10K, Marathon, and Speed Workout
- Warm-up 10 - 20 minutes to include dynamic stretches and jogging
- 5 - 8 X 800 @ 5K Pace with 1'30" RI
- 5 - 10 minute cool down, stretch

Purpose: With a break of 1'30" you get to catch your breath, but don't get the full recovery. If you feel a bit queasy when you finish your hard laps, be sure to walk a little while you wait for the time to pass. You are only doing 8 of these, however, so give each set your best.

Today's date _____

Amount of time for total workout _____

Your personal goals for this work out:

Comments:

"If you always do what you've always done, you'll always get what you've always got." Doug Kaufmann

Run Faster Workout 74

Hardest

Base Building and Strength Workout
- Warm-up 10 - 20 minutes to include dynamic stretches and jogging
- Striders for 50 yards X 3
- 10 pushups, 1 lap all out
- 20 squats, 1 lap all out
- 30 zombie kicks, 1 lap all out
- 40 leg swings, 1 lap all out
- 50 calf raises, 1 lap easy
- Repeat as far as you can get
- 5 - 10 minute cool down, stretch

Purpose: Cross training, strength training, and even just varying workouts makes your body happy. This can be done at different times during your training phases with more intensity as you get in better shape.

Today's date _____

Amount of time for total workout _____

Your personal goals for this work out:

Comments:

"It is a rough road that leads to the heights of greatness." -   Seneca

Run Faster Workout 75

Least Hard –Bonus Workout

- Veg out track workout with a twist
- Face the opposite direction on the track. Head clock-wise
- Set the music, earphones in 1 ear please, and stay in the outside lane
- Just keep moving for 30 – 60 min
- Keep your eyes open
- Move if someone is coming at you. Officially the track is used in a counter-clockwise direction
- Stretch
- Enjoy!

Purpose: Sometimes it just doesn't come together. If you've got the where-with-all to show up at the track, go for an easy, continuous workout. I guarantee you will feel better afterward.

Today's date _____

Amount of time for total workout _____

Your personal goals for this work out:

Comments:

99

The Last Word

About these Workouts

I hope you will use this book for many years to come and find improved speed and confidence in your running. Go for it! – Coach

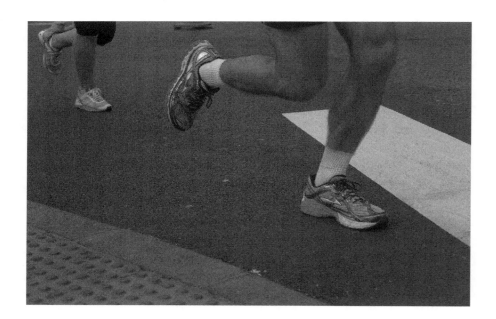

Resources

Go WOW Team – Run Walk Club Website founded by Coach Stephanie
www.gowowteam.com

Facebook – post your questions for Coach Stephanie at Go WOW Team
www.facebook.com/gowowteam

Run Better Race Faster – **Book 2** (Kindle Version) of the Live Fit Series by
Coach Stephanie **http://amzn.to/Wi5Qfg**

Run Faster Race Even Better (Kindle Version) **http://amzn.to/13s2jzl**

Coach Stephanie is **Bay Area Women's Fitness Writer** for examiner.com.
Follow her at http://tinyurl.com/ltxhftp

Gymboss Interval Timer
http://tinyurl.com/m2s76v8

Be a Better Runner by Sally Edwards, Carl Foster, PhD, FACSM, Roy M
Wallack http://amzn.to/11ZQhMM

Born to Run by Christopher McDougall http://amzn.to/WqSQDS

Author Bio
Stephanie Atwood
Go WOW Team! – Fit Women of the World

"Stephanie sure knows her stuff! Great workout...! -" Sara

"...a great coach that kicks your butt and takes care of you!" – Elke

"You meet appropriate challenges." - Melanie

Stephanie Atwood, M.A. is nationally certified as a long distance running coach through U S Track and Field (Level 2) and Road Runners Club of America. She has coached runners to numerous person bests along with Boston Marathon Qualifying Times.

She also holds certificates as a personal trainer and sports nutrition consultant and is co-founder of the Get Fit Lose Fat Eat Lots Program, utilizing metabolic eating and training techniques to increase a runner's ability to burn fat. Her **bestselling** books **Belly Fat Blowout** and **Belly Fat Blowout 2** have utilized this concept and helped numerous participants lose inches and become more efficient athletes.

Atwood has been coaching professionally and competing for more than 30 years. She ran the half mile, mile, and 2 mile in college, making it to state level. Atwood qualified for The Boston Marathon in 1976 and again in 2012. She was also a member of the first American Women's Team to climb Annapurna in the Himalayas.

In 2007 Coach Stephanie founded the running club Go WOW Team to bring coaching, camaraderie, successful training, and fitness, as a lifestyle, to adult women at all levels of ability.

Stephanie believes strongly in the "hands-on" approach to learning. "I have seen incredible things happen when an individual overcomes obstacles through her/his own effort. With some direction and encouragement from me and the team, people realize their own potential and then there's no stopping them. People are transformed and liberated by conquering their own hidden barriers. I've seen it so many times. It's wonderful teaching/supporting in this way."

Coach Stephanie has a BA in Experiential Education with a focus on bio-mechanics and kinesiology and an M.A in Communications. She is the Bay Area Women's Fitness Writer for examiner.com and coaches the Best Run Club in the Bay Area, as voted by ABC7, **Go WOW Team**.

Contact The Coach at the resources listed above, at the email address go@gowowteam.com or call 510 261-8671.

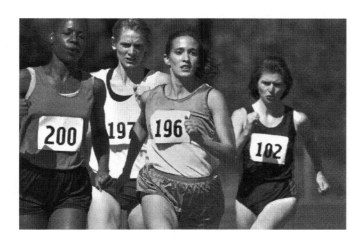

Made in the USA
Middletown, DE
23 May 2017